THA

CO

Consumables and Lifestyle
Suggestions For Nutritional
Thalassemia Management

Dr. ATHENA ABELL

1

Table of Contents

CHAPTER ONE

Introduction

Individuals who have thalassemia, a hereditary blood disorder that impacts the synthesis of hemoglobin, encounter distinctive obstacles.

As one explores the complex realm of thalassemia, it becomes apparent that a comprehensive strategy, encompassing appropriate nutritional control, is crucial for improving the overall well-being of those afflicted with this disorder.

Comprehension Of Thalassemia

Thalassemia is a hereditary condition distinguished by a disruption in the biosynthesis of hemoglobin, the critical protein accountable for oxygen transportation within erythrocytes.

Anemia ensues due to the inadequate synthesis of regular hemoglobin, a consequence of this genetic mutation. Potential complications include fatigue, frailty, and organ impairment. Thalassemia exhibits variability in severity, necessitating periodic blood transfusions for certain individuals while others are capable of managing the condition with reduced intervention.

The integration of nutritional management into the overall care of individuals with thalassemia is of the utmost importance. In light of the potential ramifications and the influence on holistic well-being, adhering to a balanced diet transcends mere discretion and becomes an imperative.

Adequate nutrition plays a crucial role in thalassemia management, including the maintenance of sufficient energy, support for the immune system, and resolution of specific complications like iron excess.

Iron-Related Thalassemia

Difficulties and Factors to Be Considered: The regulation of iron, an indispensable nutrient for the body, assumes paramount importance in the context of thalassemia. Frequent blood transfusions, which are a prevalent component of thalassemia management, result in an excessive buildup of iron within the organism. An excess of iron, a medical condition characterized by organ injury that primarily impacts the heart and liver, can occur.

Iron management in individuals with thalassemia necessitates a nuanced approach. While it is crucial for individuals to ensure adequate iron levels for essential physiological processes, it is equally important to prevent the adverse consequences associated with excessive iron. The maintenance of this intricate balance requires vigilant observation and cooperation between medical practitioners and individuals afflicted with thalassemia.

CHAPTER TWO

How To Construct A Thalassemia-Friendly Diet

Development of a thalassemia-friendly diet necessitates careful deliberation of dietary requirements and possible obstacles.

The subsequent elements are essential in establishing a dietary regimen that promotes the health and wellness of those who have thalassemia:

1. Sufficient Iron Intake: Although an excess of iron may present a

hazard, it is imperative for individuals with thalassemia to maintain adequate iron levels. Iron-dense foods, including fortified cereals, lean proteins, and legumes, can help ensure adequate iron consumption without exacerbating the risk of iron excess. Nevertheless, it is critical to seek guidance from healthcare experts in order to ascertain individualized iron needs.

2. Foods Rich in Calcium: The presence of calcium in the diet significantly reduces the adverse effects of iron absorption. Iron levels can be effectively managed by incorporating dairy products,

leafy greens, and fortified plant-based alternatives into one's diet. Supplemental calcium may be advised in accordance with individual requirements.

3. Vitamin C Supplementation: The assimilation of non-heme iron derived from plant sources is enhanced by vitamin C. By integrating citrus fruits, strawberries, and bell peppers into one's diet, iron assimilation can be enhanced without excessive dependence on animal-based sources.

4. Folate is an essential mineral for the synthesis of red blood cells;

therefore, individuals diagnosed with thalassemia may find nourishment in foods abundant in folate, including legumes, fortified cereals, and verdant vegetables. However, supplementation may be required; therefore, it is vital to consult with healthcare professionals.

5. Restrictions Regarding Iron-Enhancing Foods: Specific compounds, including the tannins present in coffee and tea, have the potential to impede the absorption of iron. By regulating the intake of these substances, particularly during meals, one can enhance the

assimilation of iron from food sources.

6. Consistent Observation and Modification: Dietary regimens for individuals with thalassemia may necessitate periodic adjustments as their nutritional requirements may progress. Consistent monitoring of iron levels and continuous communication with healthcare professionals are essential for maintaining a diet that is specifically designed to meet the unique health needs of each individual.

In summary, effectively managing thalassemia necessitates a

comprehensive strategy, with nutritional control emerging as a fundamental component in fostering holistic health. A thalassemia-friendly diet serves as more than just a means of sustenance; it empowers individuals to take an active role in their health journey.

As the intricacies of thalassemia and its nutritional subtleties are elucidated, the necessity for individuals, healthcare professionals, and nutritionists to work together becomes increasingly apparent.

By cultivating consciousness, comprehension, and a dedication to individualized attention, it is possible to enable individuals impacted by thalassemia to adopt a more salubrious and beneficial existence.

CHAPTER THREE

Foods Rich In Iron For Thalassemia

Thalassemia, a hereditary hematological disorder, presents distinct obstacles for affected individuals who must navigate their day-to-day activities with an increased consciousness of their dietary requirements.

A critical element in the management of thalassemia entails guaranteeing a sufficient consumption of iron, a mineralessential for the synthesis of red blood cells. Iron-rich food consumption is a crucial dietary strategy for those who have been diagnosed with thalassemia.

Lean meats, poultry, and fish are among the most iron-dense foods that are okay for those with thalassemia. These animal-derived sources supply heme iron, which is the most readily assimilated form of iron by the body.

Red meat, including lamb and beef, can be a delectable and effective method to increase iron levels when incorporated into meals. Moreover, in addition to enhancing iron consumption, fish such as salmon and tuna also supply omega-3 fatty acids, which are crucial for the cardiovascular system and must be taken into account by individuals with thalassemia.

It is essential for vegetarians and vegans to consume iron sources derived from plants. Legumes, including chickpeas and lentils, are commendable options due to their provision of non-heme iron in addition to fiber. Additionally, dark leafy greens such as kale and spinach provide a nutrient-dense iron boost. It is noteworthy that the absorption of non-heme iron is comparatively slower than that of heme iron; therefore, supplementing these plant-based sources with foods abundant in vitamin C can improve absorption.

Techniques Of Preparation For Iron Absorption

In addition to food selection, the manner in which iron-rich foods are prepared can influence iron absorption. The utilization of cooking methods greatly influences the body's capacity to assimilate iron from its food. For example, the addition of acidic components such as vinegar or citrus juices to meals improves the assimilation of non-heme iron.

Cast-iron cookware is an additional pragmatic approach. Small quantities of iron can be infused into meals prepared in cast-iron vessels that are acidic or high in moisture, thereby contributing to the daily iron requirement. Nevertheless, it is critical to exercise caution regarding the possibility of excessive iron absorption, especially for individuals who are enduring iron accumulation as a result of regular blood transfusions.

Preparation Of Meals For Thalassemia

In order to maintain a balanced and nutritious diet while managing thalassemia, effective meal planning is essential. A comprehensive dietary regimen for individuals diagnosed with thalassemia ought to comprise a variety of foods that are abundant in vitamin C, iron, and other vital nutrients.

Breakfast choices may comprise cereals fortified with fruits, thereby offering the added advantages of iron and vitamin C. Lean meats, poultry, or plant-based proteins such as tofu or legumes may be combined with vitamin C-rich vegetables for lunch and supper.

It is imperative to maintain a harmonious proportion of protein consumption with other vital nutrients, including folate, vitamin B12, and zinc, all of which are indispensable in bolstering the overall well-being of individuals afflicted with thalassemia.

CHAPTER FOUR

Ideas For Snacks And Quick Bites

Snacks that are nutritious are vital for sustaining energy levels throughout the day, particularly for those with thalassemia who are susceptible to fatigue. Snacks that are ideal should be both convenient and nourishing. Nuts and seeds are commendable alternatives due to their provision of healthful lipids and iron. Moreover, dried fruits, including raisins and apricots, can provide a delicious and iron-rich substitute.

Berry-topped Greek yogurt is a satiety-inducing, protein-rich refreshment that is also an excellent source of vitamin C and dairy. Individuals who prefer piquant foods may find hummus accompanied by whole-grain crackers or raw vegetables to be a gratifying texture in addition to enhancing their iron consumption.

Caffeine Suitable For Thalassemia

Maintaining adequate hydration is of utmost importance for all individuals, but those with thalassemia may also benefit nutritionally from the beverages they select. Beverages that are high in iron can serve as a suitable accompaniment to meals and refreshments. In particular, fortified fruit beverages that are rich in vitamin C can serve as a beneficial supplement to one's dietary regimen.

Herbal infusions formulated with dandelion or nettle, which are abundant in iron, offer a palatable and healthful substitute. It is also critical to maintain a watchful eye on caffeine consumption, as an excess of this substance can impede the absorption of iron. Choosing water infused with citrus slices or caffeine-free herbal beverages can provide dual benefits of increased hydration and enhanced iron absorption.

As summary, effectively managing thalassemia via nutrition necessitates careful preparation and an emphasis on integrating foods abundant in iron into a nutritionally balanced dietary regimen. By acquiring knowledge about the intricacies of iron assimilation, employing strategic culinary methods, and integrating a variety of nutrient-rich foods into their diet, individuals diagnosed with thalassemia can proactively foster their general health and welfare. By incorporating delectable meal options, nutritious munchies, and conscientious beverage selections, individuals with thalassemia can embark on a voyage of holistic and empowering body nourishment.

The Use Of Flavorful Herbs And Spices To Improve Flavor Without Negating Nutrition

The culinary practice of incorporating herbs and seasonings not only enhances the gustatory experience but also improves the nutritional composition of dishes. When dietary restrictions are of the utmost importance, as in the case of thalassemia, the prudent application of aromatic herbs and seasonings becomes critical.

Specific herbs and spices, including garlic, ginger, and turmeric, are renowned not only for their potent flavors but also for their anti-inflammatory characteristics, which may prove beneficial for thalassemia patients who suffer from chronic inflammation. Basil, mint, and cilantro are examples of herbs that impart vital nutrients to dishes while also imparting a sense of freshness.

By harmonizing flavors with seasonings and spices, thalassemia-friendly dishes are enriched with anti-inflammatory and antioxidant compounds, which positively impact the general health of those who are thalassemia-managing.

Particular Considerations Regarding Thalassemia In Children

For optimal growth and development, children with thalassemia necessitate particular care to ensure that their nutritional requirements are adequately addressed. It is imperative to consume a sufficient quantity of iron-rich foods, including lean meats, legumes, and fortified cereals, due to the intrinsic difficulties that thalassemia presents in terms of iron metabolism.

Furthermore, it is frequently the case that children diagnosed with thalassemia necessitate a dietary regimen that is not only rich in essential nutrients but also customized to suit their individual preferences. By integrating an assortment of flavors and textures into their meals, diners can enhance their overall dining experience and be more inclined to adhere to dietary recommendations.

Ensuring that children with thalassemia have access to a positive and supportive food environment is largely the responsibility of their parents and caregivers. Consistent surveillance of nutritional status, in conjunction with healthcare professionals, guarantees that any insufficiencies are expeditiously attended to, thereby promoting healthy development and overall well-being.

CHAPTER FIVE

Recipes For Meals Suitable For Thalassemia

The preparation of thalassemia-friendly dishes necessitates a deliberative approach to ingredient choice and culinary methodology. It is crucial to include iron-rich foods in one's diet, including spinach, lentils, and lean poultry. The incorporation of whole cereals, such as quinoa and brown rice, into a diet enhances nutritional content and guarantees a consistent supply of energy.

Illustrative cuisine may comprise:

1.Soup of Spinach and Lentils Enhanced with Iron:

• Components: spinach, lentils, tomatoes, garlic, and a combination of herbs and seasonings that are healthy for thalassemia.

• Method: By simmering lentils and vegetables with aromatic seasonings, a nourishing and delectable broth is produced that is also rich in nutrients.

2.Quinoa salad dressed with citrus juice:

• Quinoa, an assortment of vegetables, citrus fruits, and a delicate citrus vinaigrette are the components.

• Approach: Incorporate cooked quinoa alongside an assortment of vibrant vegetables and a piquant citrus vinaigrette to create a nourishing and invigorating supper.

Sweets And Desserts Featuring A Nutritional Twist

Dessert consumption is not necessarily forbidden for those with thalassemia. Desserts can be both delectable and health-promoting by integrating ingredients that are rich in nutrients.

Consider the following dessert options:

1.Greek yogurt parfait with berries:

• Greek yogurt and a variety of fruit arranged in tiers, adorned with a scattering of almonds.

• This delicacy is rich in protein and antioxidants and possesses a sweet and sour taste.

2.Skewers of dark chocolate-dipped fruit:

• Fresh fruit skewers that have been coated in dark chocolate.

When consumed in moderation, dark chocolate can serve as a source of antioxidants and iron, rendering it both a pleasurable and nourishing indulgence.

Dining Out While Having Thalassemia: Suggestions And Mechanisms

In order to maintain a thalassemia-friendly diet while dining out, communication and strategic planning are required. Some helpful suggestions include:

1.Menu Preparation in Advance:

When selecting restaurants, give preference to those that offer a varied selection of menu items that cater to individuals with thalassemia.

2.Interactions with the Restaurant Staff:

Communication with the staff regarding dietary restrictions and requests for modifications guarantees that meals are in accordance with the specific requirements of thalassemia.

3.When Selecting Steamed and Grilled Options:

Selecting grilled or broiled dishes over frying reduces the incorporation of added lipids while preserving the authentic tastes of the ingredients.

4.Carrying Snacks Suitable for Thalassemia Patients:

The availability of portable munchies that are high in nutrients serves as a dietary supplement between meals, thereby discouraging the desire to eat less nutritious alternatives.

In summary, adopting a gastronomic approach that is accommodating to individuals with thalassemia necessitates a

symphonious fusion of savory seasonings and herbs, astuteness towards the needs of children, laboriously designed recipes, nourishing deserts, and calculated approaches to dining out. By integrating these components into their everyday routines, individuals with thalassemia can enjoy a varied and enlightening gastronomic encounter while placing their health and wellbeing first.

CHAPTER SIX

Creative Hydration Ideas And The Importance Of Staying Hydrated

Water, which is considered the "elixir of life," is indispensable for the maintenance of health and well-being. Maintaining sufficient hydration is critical for a multitude of physiological processes, including temperature regulation, digestion, and nutrient assimilation. In the context of thalassemia, a hereditary blood disorder distinguished by inadequate production of

hemoglobin, the importance of hydration is heightened.

It is imperative that individuals with thalassemia maintain adequate hydration, as it aids in the mitigation of certain symptoms that are linked to the condition. Thalassemia patients frequently encounter fatigue and frailty, both of which can be worsened by dehydration. Moreover, maintaining adequate hydration prevents complications associated with blood circulation, thereby promoting optimal body function.

In order to ensure adequate hydration, it is advised that a minimum of eight 8-ounce containers of water be consumed daily. Nonetheless, inventive approaches to hydration can improve the variety and enjoyment of this routine. As an illustration, infused water imparts a delightful surge of flavor devoid of any artificial ingredients or added carbohydrates. Engage in the exploration of various fruit, herb, and vegetable combinations in order to craft customized, invigorating concoctions.

Vitamin C And Thalassemia: Improving Iron Absorption

Thalassemia frequently induces iron overload as a consequence of recurrent blood transfusions, potentially giving rise to organ dysfunction and other complications. On the other hand, vitamin C can facilitate the absorption of iron from dietary sources. Consuming foods that are abundant in vitamin C is a straightforward and efficacious method to enhance the absorption of iron and promote general well-being.

Broccoli, citrus fruits, strawberries, and bell peppers are all rich in vitamin C. To optimize the assimilation of non-heme iron, which is present in plant-based foods and supplements, contemplate integrating the following foods into your meal or refreshment routine. The interdependence of vitamin C and iron highlights the criticality of thalassemia patients adhering to a well-planned and balanced diet.

Lifestyle Suggestions For Nutritional Thalassemia Management

In addition to hydration and strategic nutrient coupling, the management of thalassemia via nutrition necessitates the adoption of a comprehensive and conscientious dietary philosophy. Here are some opinions for a healthy lifestyle:

1.A balanced diet is one in which a variety of nutrient-dense foods are consumed. Consume fruits, vegetables, lean proteins, and whole grains to ensure that your

body receives the necessary vitamins and minerals.

2.Supplementation: Consult with healthcare professionals in close collaboration to ascertain the necessity of any particular vitamin or mineral supplements. Supplementary support in the form of folic acid, vitamin D, or other relevant substances may be necessary to mitigate potential deficiencies associated with thalassemia.

3.Thoracocytes are critically ill patients who must undergo routine blood tests and health examinations. Continual

monitoring of critical health indicators, including hemoglobin levels, iron status, and overall nutritional health, facilitates prompt interventions and modifications to the treatment regimen.

4.It is crucial to consistently maintain adequate levels of hydration. Establish a daily water consumption objective and devise inventive methods to achieve it, including consuming hydrating foods like cantaloupe, infusing water with natural flavors, and imbibing medicinal beverages.

5.Adopting a mindful dining practice can assist in cultivating a constructive rapport with food. Supporting overall well-being requires paying attention to appetite and satiety indicators, savoring the flavors of each meal, and being mindful of portion sizes.

Conclusion

In summary, the complex interaction among nutrition, thalassemia, and hydration emphasizes the importance of adopting a comprehensive approach to health administration. Adequate hydration is not a trivial habit, but rather a fundamental

aspect of overall health, particularly for those who are managing the difficulties associated with thalassemia. In addition to recognizing the significance of vitamin C in facilitating iron assimilation, innovative hydration strategies contribute to a comprehensive approach to managing this genetic blood disorder.

Lifestyle recommendations for nutrition-based thalassemia management emphasize the importance of a diverse and well-balanced diet, individualized supplementation when required, consistent monitoring of health

indicators, and the development of mindful eating practices. By adopting these principles, individuals diagnosed with thalassemia can enhance their ability to lead satisfying lives, alleviate the consequences of the disorder, and maximize their general well-being and energy.